P9-EES-134

Frequently Asked Questions

all about
coenzyme Q10

RAY SAHELIAN, MD

AVERY PUBLISHING GROUP
Garden City Park • New York

The information contained in this book is based upon the research and personal and professional experiences of the author. They are not intended as a substitute for consulting with your physician or other health care provider. Any attempt to diagnose and treat an illness should be done under the direction of a health care professional.

The publisher does not advocate the use of any particular health care protocol, but believes the information in this book should be available to the public. The publisher and author are not responsible for any adverse effects or consequences resulting from the use of any of the suggestions, preparations, or procedures discussed in this book. Should the reader have any questions concerning the appropriateness of any procedure or preparation mentioned, the author and the publisher strongly suggest consulting a professional health care advisor.

Series cover designer: Eric Macaluso
Cover image courtesy of Barry Axelrod Studios, Inc.

ISBN: 0-89529-904-6

Copyright 1998 © by Ray Sahelian, M.D.

Printed in the United States of America

10   9   8   7   6   5   4   3   2   1

Contents

Introduction

"Why didn't my cardiologist tell me about CoQ_{10}?" Racquel asked me. "Ever since I've been on it, I'm not short of breath anymore. I can get all the housework done without having to sit down and rest."

Racquel, a grandmother, is seventy-five years of age. She had a triple bypass heart operation in 1992 and couldn't return to full health after the surgery. At least once a month, she'd get a mild episode of angina, or heart pain. And her constant state of low-energy had taken away her excitement about life. Then, I recommended that she try coenzyme Q_{10}, commonly referred to as CoQ_{10}. It changed her life.

"I felt the benefits the second day that I took the 30 mg pill," she said. "I'm surprised more doctors don't know about CoQ_{10}."

When Racquel finished her bottle of CoQ_{10}, it took only two days for her to feel that, once again, something was missing. Her fatigue came back, and Racquel spent most of her time sitting around the house. So she purchased more CoQ$_{10}$ and resumed supplementation. The benefits returned almost immediately.

Racquel's story is an example of how significantly CoQ$_{10}$ can benefit the individual who suffers from heart disease. You probably know that heart disease is the most common cause of death in the United States. In recent years, researchers have discovered the important roles that diet, some vitamins (such as vitamin E and the B vitamins), and certain vitamin-like nutrients play in keeping the heart healthy. Unfortunately, most medical doctors still do not recommend these helpful substances to their patients, and CoQ$_{10}$ goes largely unnoticed.

CoQ$_{10}$ is one of the most important nutrients for your heart—and one of the most overlooked. In *All About Coenzyme Q$_{10}$*, you'll learn about how this remarkable vitamin-like substance can strengthen your heart and reduce your risk of cardiovascular disease. And to give you the necessary background to understand these benefits, a whole chapter is dedicated to explaining cardiovascular disease. You'll also learn about CoQ$_{10}$'s many other potential benefits. For example, it is helpful in the prevention of recurrent breast cancer; may help coun-ter gingivitis; and serves as a natural energizer, possibly combating chronic fatigue. I'll provide instruction on how to go about supplementing with CoQ$_{10}$ on a daily basis. There's also a helpful Suggested Readings list at the back of this book. By the time you finish reading *All About Coenzyme Q₁₀*, you'll be convinced that this nutrient is one of the most important supplements you could, and should, take.

1.

The ABCs of Coenzyme Q_{10}

Due to its rather technical name and rather recently recognized potential, coenzyme Q_{10}, commonly referred to as CoQ_{10}, can be quite intimidating. So this chapter explains exactly what this substance is, and what it can do for your body.

Q. What exactly is CoQ_{10}?

A. CoQ_{10} is also known to scientists as ubiquinol. It is a naturally occurring nutrient normally present in every cell in the body, and also available through foods (especially fish and meats, particularly organ meats). The body makes CoQ_{10}, but many people probably don't make it very well, due to the highly complicated biochemical process required for its production. CoQ_{10} is also sold as a dietary supplement at vitamin stores, pharmacies, retail outlets, and through mail order companies.

As we age, the body loses its efficiency in manufacturing important nutrients. In addition, people with serious diseases (such as heart disease and cancer) tend to have low CoQ$_{10}$ levels. Hence, even though the young may be able to get enough CoQ$_{10}$ by making it and ingesting it through diet, a gradual deficiency may develop as we get to our middle age and older years. Thus, supplementation can prove beneficial.

Q. Is CoQ$_{10}$ a vitamin?

A. A vitamin is defined as any nutrient that cannot be manufactured by the body (at least not in sufficient amounts) and hence has to be ingested through foods. CoQ$_{10}$ is technically not a true vitamin, since the body has the ability to manufacture it. Thus, it is referred to as a vitamin-like nutrient. Nevertheless, there are many instances in which the body may not be able to produce sufficient CoQ$_{10}$. In such cases, supplements can offer tremendous health benefits. Interestingly, when the late Karl Folkers, Ph.D. (one of the pioneering CoQ$_{10}$ researchers) was in his eighties, he acknowledged that he was involved in the naming of CoQ$_{10}$ and that he regretted not calling it a vitamin.

Q. What does CoQ$_{10}$ do in the body?

A. This important nutrient plays two major roles in the body. First, CoQ$_{10}$ helps in the energy production within each cell. The body, just like a car, needs fuel. Our primary source of fuel is through fats, proteins, and carbohydrates in the diet. After digestion in the stomach, the nutrients from foodstuffs are absorbed into the bloodstream and circulate to various tissues and cells. The cells have to break down the sugars, fats, and amino acids in a form that makes energy. This energy production occurs in organelles, or microscopic organ-like structures, called *mitochondria*, and CoQ$_{10}$ plays a key role in this activity.

There are hundreds, sometimes thousands, of mitochondria within each cell. In a sense, they are the factories of your cells, with the final product being energy. The energy that is produced is stored in a chemical called *adenosine triphosphate*, or simply *ATP*. It is carried by electrons and protons, which are subatomic particles. Numerous compounds are responsible for moving these energetic electrons and protons around in cells. CoQ$_{10}$ is one of these compounds. Others include the B vitamins, carnitine, and alpha-lipoic acid.

CoQ$_{10}$ also serves as an antioxidant, which is its

second role. By controlling the movement of electrons, CoQ$_{10}$ limits the production of dangerous *free radicals*, which are molecules lacking one electron in what should be a pair. Antioxidants are considered to be anti-cancerous. Read on for more detail.

Q. What are free radicals?

A. During normal metabolism, or processing, of foodstuffs and while fighting infections, the body produces unstable molecules or atoms that can damage cells. These destructive molecules are called free radicals; they generally consist of an unstable oxygen atom missing an electron. Atoms, such as hydrogen and oxygen, usually have a pair of electrons spinning around them. When one of these electrons is lost, the atom can then steal an electron from a neighboring molecule that is part of a healthy cell. This process can create havoc and damage.

The body has ways to detoxify these free radicals, and there's often a good balance between oxidation (free-radical activity) and antioxidation (neutralizing of free radicals). In fact, your body normally produces powerful natural antioxidants that help fight these free radicals (sometimes called *oxidants*). You obtain additional antioxidants by eating a lot of fruits and vegetables or by taking sup-

plements. But when a shift occurs leading to a pre-
ponderance of oxidation without adequate antioxidant support, the body undergoes what's called
oxidative stress.

Cigarette smoke, fried foods, ozone, excessive
sun exposure, car exhaust, certain drugs, radiation,
and air pollution are common sources of free radicals. The continuing exposure to oxidants takes a
toll on the body, resulting in specific changes in
cells. These changes include damage to fatty acids,
inactivation of enzymes, deterioration of cell mem-
branes, breakdown of proteins, and damage to
DNA (deoxyribonucleic acid, which contains
instructions for how cells should behave). For
example, if free radicals damage DNA, the eventu-
al consequence could be a higher likelihood of cancer. If the damage occurs in arteries that supply
blood to the heart, it could eventually lead to hardening of the arteries and heart attack.

Q. How does CoQ₁₀ function as an antioxidant to fight free radicals?

A. The chemical structure of CoQ_{10} allows it to easily accept electrons and also give up electrons. Giving
up electrons helps to stabilize or "quench" free radicals. Furthermore, in the bloodstream, CoQ_{10} is main-
ly transported by lipoproteins such as LDLs (low-

density lipoproteins) and HDLs (high-density lipoproteins). Lipoproteins also carry and transport cholesterol through the bloodstream. The free radical
attack of LDLs—the oxidation of LDLs or the cholesterol in them—leads to damage and the building up
of plaques in the arteries. Some researchers believe
that CoQ$_{10}$ is the first antioxidant to be depleted
when LDLs are attacked by free radicals, so we know
that its use is priority in such a situation.

Many antioxidants work together in preserving
each other. Therefore, a sufficient intake of CoQ$_{10}$
can help regenerate vitamin E and other antioxidants, as well. This is an important concept to keep
in mind when you plan to supplement with many
antioxidants. You will need lower doses of each
because they work synergistically.

Q. Which conditions does CoQ$_{10}$ help?

A. Research and the clinical practice of some
physicians has shown CoQ$_{10}$ to be helpful in treating a number of conditions. Among these are: congestive heart failure; coronary artery disease, appli-
cable even in cases of previous heart attack and for
those planning to have a heart operation; high cholesterol levels; high blood pressure (hypertension);
mitral valve prolapse; breast cancer; periodontitis
or gingivitis; and fatique.

CoQ$_{10}$ has been studied most thoroughly for its roles in maintaining normal heart function and preventing serious heart disease. Heart muscle is constantly using energy to pump blood through the body. CoQ$_{10}$ helps in that energy production. Dozens of well-designed and performed human trials have been published in the scientific literature regarding the heart-energizing benefits of this nutrient. Over the next few years, we may find many more medical, psychological, and neurological conditions in which this nutrient could provide benefits.

Q. When was CoQ$_{10}$ discovered, and when did it become available?

A. In 1957, Frederick Crane, Ph.D., then of the University of Wisconsin, isolated an orange substance from the mitochondria of beef heart. The following year, Folkers and coworkers at Merck, Sharpe, and Dohme synthesized CoQ$_{10}$ in the laboratory. CoQ$_{10}$ is an orange molecule, which is why many CoQ$_{10}$ supplements have this color.

This nutrient became widely available as an over-the-counter supplement in the United States in the mid-1980s. Since then, its popularity has been increasing. More individuals are recognizing the benefits of CoQ$_{10}$ and informing their doctors about it.

Q. When was CoQ$_{10}$ first used in the therapy of heart disease?

A. In 1964, seven years after the discovery of CoQ$_{10}$, a Japanese researcher became the first person in the world to demonstrate that CoQ$_{10}$ could be successfully used in the therapy of congestive heart failure, which is a very serious form of heart disease. The condition is characterized not by blockages in the arteries (although they may be present), but by a lack of energy in the heart muscle, affecting its ability to pump blood. In the 1970s, researchers discovered that CoQ$_{10}$ has antioxidant abilities, and dozens of studies on humans since then have indicated this nutrient to be safe and effective in a variety of cardiovascular conditions.

Q. Why don't more doctors know about CoQ$_{10}$?

A. Unfortunately, most doctors in practice are not familiar with the published research regarding the therapeutic potential of CoQ$_{10}$ because many of the journals they read rarely discuss the benefits of this and other nutrients. And why is that? You probably know the reason: nutrients cannot be patented and

thus are of little interest to pharmaceutical companies who advertise and sponsor the majority of the
journals read by doctors. The story is a little different in Europe and Japan, where health-care profes-
sionals already have been prescribing CoQ$_{10}$ to
patients with congestive heart failure and other
conditions for many years. In fact, CoQ$_{10}$ is the fifth
most commonly prescribed "drug" in Japan.

Q. Is there good science behind CoQ$_{10}$?

A. Hundreds of scientific studies have been published on CoQ$_{10}$, including many involving human
subjects. CoQ$_{10}$ has also been the subject of ten
international scientific and medical meetings.
Furthermore, the role of CoQ$_{10}$ in energy production was the basis of the 1978 Nobel prize in chem-
istry, awarded to the late Peter Mitchell, Ph.D., a
British researcher. All of this indicates very good
quality science behind CoQ$_{10}$.

Q. How much CoQ$_{10}$ do we get from food?

A. Dietary intake of CoQ$_{10}$ normally ranges from 2
to 20 mg a day. Most of this comes from meat and

fish consumption. The richest source of CoQ_{10} is organ meats, such as heart and liver, which relatively few people eat. Plants contain only small amounts of coenzyme Q compounds. Therefore, vegetarians may not get adequate amounts of this nutrient.

As you will read in Chapter 5, young people tend to get adequate amounts of CoQ_{10} from food and from their bodies' natural production of this nutrient. But older individuals may not manufacture CoQ_{10} well enough, or absorb it efficiently. In these cases, supplementation is wise.

2.

Understanding Cardiovascular Disease

Without the rhythmic pumping of the heart, none of us would be alive. Most of us are fortunate that, in youth, the heart and blood vessels are very healthy and we don't have to worry when we run or exert ourselves. Unfortunately, as we get older, many of us develop problems with the cardiovascular system.

The most frequent cardiovascular conditions seen by doctors are hypertension, heart failure, atherosclerosis, angina, heart attacks, arrhythmias, and strokes. Many of these conditions have similar causes, whether it be poor diet, lack of exercise, smoking, excess alcohol, psychological factors such as depression and anxiety, and/or deficiencies in nutrients. Genetics can also play a role, especially in those whose heart disease is manifested in their thirties or forties. Coenzyme Q$_{10}$ has been found to be beneficial to the heart and blood vessels. So that you can fully understand CoQ$_{10}$'s role, this chapter offers basic definitions of the types and processes of cardiovascular disease.

Q. What is hypertension?

A. Hypertension refers to elevated or high blood pressure. Generally, blood pressure is considered high when systolic blood pressure exceeds 140 and diastolic blood pressure is over 90. Systolic pressure refers to the pressure exerted on the artery wall each time the heart contracts. Diastolic pressure refers to the pressure in the artery during the brief part of a second when the heart is relaxing. Hypertension puts strain on the vessels themselves, on the heart, and on the kidneys.

Q. What is heart failure?

A. Heart failure is often called *congestive heart failure* or *CHF*. The heart is made of muscle tissue. The effects of aging, poor diet, heart attacks, stress, viral infections, smoking, and alcohol abuse weaken this muscle. Furthermore, hypertension can be a cause of heart failure because the heart has to constantly pump against a lot of resistance in the arteries. This uses up CoQ_{10} and ATP, or the cells' energy. As the heart becomes weaker and pumps less efficiently, blood and fluid can slowly backup, or congest, into the lungs and the rest of the body, leading to CHF.

The backing up of fluid in the lungs is called *pulmonary edema*, while fluid in the lower extremities is called *peripheral edema*. Doctors use the term *ejection fraction* (EF) to describe the percentage of blood pumped from the left ventricle with every heartbeat. People with healthy hearts have an ejection fraction of between 50 and 70 percent, while those with poor hearts can have an EF of as low as 30 or even 15 percent.

There are different degrees of CHF, depending on the damage to the heart muscle. Someone with a bad case of edema has trouble breathing because the fluid in the lungs takes up valuable lung space. Also, the feet become puffy. In such situations, when you push the skin on top of the feet with your finger, a clear indentation is left. Doctors often give digitalis or other drugs to improve the pumping of the heart, but such drugs often have serious side effects and do not correct the underlying problem. CoQ_{10} may be a better option.

Q. What is atherosclerosis?

A. Atherosclerosis is also known as "hardening of the arteries." Plaque formations in the walls of the arteries narrow the openings through which blood can flow. Sometimes a clot can form and block the artery, denying the supply of blood to an organ or tissue. When atherosclerosis occurs in the coronary arteries—that is, the arteries of the heart—we call this *coronary artery disease* or *CAD.* If the supply of the blood to a part of the heart muscle is completely interrupted, a *heart attack* occurs. If the blood supply is cut off to a part of the brain, a *stroke* occurs.

Q. What is angina?

A. Angina refers to chest pain, which is often caused by either a spasm in the coronary arteries or by a small blood clot that causes a temporary blockage. Patients experience temporary pressure, squeezing, or fullness in the chest. Many factors can precipitate angina, including physical or emotional stress, exposure to cold, or even eating a huge meal. When the coronary arteries are narrowed (by plaques, for example), any further constricting can significantly decrease blood flow and, therefore, oxygen supply to the heart muscle, leading to angina. Many patients with angina carry nitroglycerin tablets that they place under the tongue. Nitroglycerin helps relax the arteries.

Q. What is an arrhythmia?

A. An arrhythmia is an irregular heartbeat. The heart has four chambers, two atria and two ventricles. Atrial arrhythmias come from dysfunction in the atria, the two smaller chambers on top of the ventricles. Ventricular arrhythmias, caused by dysfunction in the ventricles, are more serious and can sometimes lead to fainting and death. Multiple factors can lead to arrhythmias. These include heart attacks; excessive stress; high dose ingestion of stimulants such as caffeine, ephedra, and amphetamines; alcohol overconsumption; certain antidepressant medications; and /or electrical abnormalities of the heart conduction system.

3.

Coenzyme Q_{10} and Cardiovascular Disease

Although the role of CoQ_{10} has been studied in a number of disorders, thus far the most obvious benefits have been found in its effects on cardiovascular disease. The heart works every second of every day, using up a lot of energy. CoQ_{10} can play a role in energy production, improving the function of heart muscle, and, thus, the cardiovascular system. Let's examine some of the research regarding the use of this nutrient in heart health.

Q. Does CoQ_{10} reduce hypertension?

A. Yes, it appears to aid in lowering blood pressure. Dr. V. Digiesi and colleagues, from the

University of Florence Medical School in Florence, Italy, enrolled twenty-six patients with hypertension in a study to determine if CoQ_{10} could influence their blood pressure. The patients were given 50 mg of CoQ_{10} twice daily for ten weeks. Between the beginning and end of supplementation, systolic blood pressure decreased from an average of 164 to 146, and diastolic blood pressure dropped from 98 to 86. These are significant and healthy decreases.

The researchers speculate that the blood pressure lowering may have been due to the ability of CoQ_{10} to decrease arterial resistance by relaxing the muscles that surround the arteries. After all, one of the causes of high blood pressure is that the walls of the arteries contract, thus preventing the relaxation of the arteries. Incidentally, in addition to these benefits, cholestrol levels in the study's participants dropped from 223 to 213.

Physicians and researchers at the Institute of Biomedical Research, University of Texas, Austin, gave CoQ_{10} to a total of 100 patients with hypertension. The dosage was not fixed but adjusted based on clinical response, generally averaging 200 mg daily. The patients were followed closely with frequent outpatient clinic visits to record blood pressure and to note overall status. A definite improvement was noted in blood pressure within the first month of therapy. Echocardiograms done to check the function of the heart showed an improvement of the left ventricular muscle tissue.

The clinical experience of physicians indicates that CoQ$_{10}$ has a role to play in lowering blood pressure. However, the hypertensive individual should not rely exclusively on this nutrient. Many other nutrients, including calcium, magnesium, and omega-3 fatty acids (fish oils) also play important roles in the management of high blood pressure. Also, a lot of additional nutritional and lifestyle advice has been provided to the public regarding approaches to treating hypertension: use your salt shaker less; eat more fiber; take potassium; lose weight; stop smoking; stop drinking alcohol; eat more fruits and vegetables; take magnesium pills; relax, and take a vacation.

Q. Should I combine CoQ$_{10}$ and other nutritional approaches with blood pressure medicines?

A. Even though CoQ$_{10}$ plays a part in reducing hypertension, it is not a cure. Other nutritional and pharmaceutical agents may be required. When hypertension does not respond to a nutritional approach alone, it is appropriate to add pharmaceutical agents. The aim should be to decrease the dosages of pharmaceutical drugs by combining them with nutritional supplements.

In cases of mild to moderate hypertension, such as a systolic blood pressure less than 170, it would be worthwhile to try nutritional approaches for a few weeks before using a drug. If it is found that medication is necessary, combining nutrients and medicines has to be done slowly and methodically. Caution advises us to start with low dosages and gradually build up. The dosage of CoQ_{10} for reducing hypertension can range from 20 to 60 mg daily.

In cases of severe hypertension, such as a systolic pressure greater than 170 or 180, a pharmaceutical agent may have to be used initially, until a patient begins to improve lifestyle habits. If you are in this position, your doctor can recommend one of several antihypertensive medicines. Then, once you reduce your blood pressure to a healthy level, you can work with your physician in order to combine pharmaceuticals with a natural approach.

Q. Does CoQ_{10} help in heart failure?

A. The best studied aspect of CoQ_{10} therapy is its role in helping patients in improving their cardiac function. Numerous published studies have shown that CoQ_{10} plays a significant therapeutic role in treating congestive heart failure. In fact, researchers applied a *meta-analysis* to eight controlled clinical trials of CoQ$_{10}$-treatment of congestive heart failure. A meta-analysis means that the results of all previously published studies are pooled together and then statistically reviewed. This review revealed a significant improvement in several important cardiac functions.

"In patients with chronic heart failure, the addition of CoQ$_{10}$ to conventional therapy reduces the hospitalization rate for worsening of heart failure and the incidence of serious cardiovascular complications," wrote Dr. C. Morisco of the University of Degli Studi Federico, Naples, Italy. In a well-controlled study, Morisco and colleagues gave six patients 50 mg of CoQ$_{10}$ three times a day for four weeks. It was concluded that the administration of CoQ$_{10}$ significantly improved the amount of blood the heart pumped at each stroke.

I believe CoQ$_{10}$ supplementation should be the first action doctors recommend when a patient's heart is not pumping properly. CoQ$_{10}$ supplements would hopefully decrease the requirements of other medicines, such as digitalis, ACE inhibitors, and other drugs used to manage CHF. Or, perhaps, the addition of CoQ$_{10}$ would decrease the dosage required of other medicines.

Q. What's the appropriate dosage to treat CHF?

A. Since each patient is unique, it's difficult to give dosage recommendations that would apply to everyone. However, a safe way would be to start at 30 mg daily, and gradually increase this dose over the next few weeks to obtain the desired clinical effect. I strongly recommend supervision by a health-care provider, particularly if you are taking another heart drug. The maximum dosage should generally not exceed 120 mg daily, unless your doctor believes higher dosages used temporarily could provide you with more benefits. There are patients who need as much as 200 mg of CoQ_{10} daily.

It is best to split your dosage. If you're planning to take 60 mg per day, take 30 mg in the morning and 30 mg with lunch. Some people report feeling a little too energized at night and find they have difficulty sleeping if they take CoQ_{10} past noon.

Q. Is CoQ_{10} the only nutrient that can reduce my risk of heart failure?

A. No. An additional nutrient to consider is L-carnitine, at about 1 g a day. Carnitine helps transport long-chain fatty acids across the mitochondrial membrane and helps with energy production. Studies involving athletes have shown that carnitine supplementation can even improve aerobic performance. So it has a significant influence on energy production. You'll find more information on this in Chapter 5.

Q. Does CoQ$_{10}$ combat atherosclerosis?

A. The process of plaque formation in the walls of arteries is complicated and involves many factors, including oxidation and inflammation. When there's a lack of adequate antioxidants present in the blood, some substances, such as low-density lipoproteins (LDLs), can oxidize and damage the lining of the arteries. This creates an inflammatory reaction, leading to the initiation of atherosclerosis.

Among other roles, CoQ$_{10}$ protects the lipoproteins—in the bloodstream from being oxidized. In fact, at least one study done at the Heart Research Institute in Sidney, Australia, has shown that CoQ$_{10}$ may be a better antioxidant in terms of lipoprotein protection than vitamin E. So, as an antioxidant, CoQ$_{10}$ can reduce the risk of atherosclerosis.

Keep in mind that there are dozens of important antioxidants in the body and in our foods which also play crucial roles in preventing atherosclerosis. These include vitamins C and E; the flavonoids and carotenoids found in fruits, vegetables, and herbs; the nutrients alpha-lipoic acid and N-acetylcysteine; and others. Therefore, even though CoQ_{10} is an important antioxidant, we shouldn't over-emphasize its importance at the expense of the other antioxidants.

Also remember that CoQ_{10} and additional antioxidants are *part* of the solution, not the entire solution. Atherosclerosis has multiple causes. The most common are smoking, stress, excess alcohol, and eating calorie-dense processed foods. High levels of *homocysteine*, a substance made from the amino acid methionine, can be a significant factor. The use of B vitamins, particularly folic acid, B_6, and B_{12}, can help reduce levels of homocysteine. Another nutrient that can help reduce homocysteine levels is *betaine*, also known as *TMG* (trimethylglycine). In addition, healthy lifestyle habits are essential.

Q. What is a recommended dosage for CoQ_{10} in the prevention of atherosclerosis?

A. The dosage of CoQ_{10} that I recommend for its work as an antioxidant is 30 mg daily. I don't see a reason to take more, since I suggest taking many other antioxidants along with CoQ_{10}. Please keep in mind that many antioxidants work together. Therefore, I recommend that you also take vitamins C and E, and that you consume a good number of antioxidants through fresh produce. Additional antioxidants to consider include alpha-lipoic acid and carnitine (or its acetyl-L-carnitine form).

Q. What can I do if I have high cholesterol levels?

A. If you have high cholesterol levels, your health-care practitioner may recommend that you start lifestyle changes that will decrease these levels. Many doctors will prescribe cholesterol-lowering drugs. These drugs are controversial; many of the results have been mixed. For example, a certain type of cholesterol-lowering drugs called *statins* interfere with your body's production of CoQ_{10} and could actually be harmful to heart muscle.

In a 1996 study conducted in France, forty patients with high cholesterol levels were given statin drugs and compared to an untreated group. The ones who received the statin drugs had lower levels of blood CoQ_{10} and showed evidence of mito-chondrial (or energy-production) dysfunction.

Statins are a double-edged sword, and the above finding is certainly an area of concern to patients who are prescribed this class of drugs.

Before resorting to drugs, I generally prefer to use natural methods to lower cholesterol levels. Actually, protecting cholesterol from being oxidized by free radicals is as important as trying to lower its level. Most patients respond well to natural therapies. These include: increasing intake of fresh foods, such as fruits and vegetables; lowering caloric intake by eating fewer sweets and fatty foods; increasing fiber intake (such as psyllium fiber); adding fish to the diet or taking fish oil capsules; engaging in mild to moderate exercise; and taking supplements, especially antioxidants. CoQ$_{10}$ should be among the supplements.

Q. How does CoQ$_{10}$ influence angina and heart attacks?

A. It's likely to reduce your risk of having these problems. Remember, CoQ$_{10}$ protects your arteries from oxidative damage, which leads to plaque accumulations. If the arteries that supply blood and oxygen to your heart are clogged up with plaque, then you have coronary artery disease with a high risk for a heart attack. It now becomes easy for a clot to form in these narrowed arteries, leading to a sudden blockage of blood and oxygen supply to the muscles of the heart. If you've already had a heart attack, unless you've made some drastic dietary and lifestyle habit changes, your odds of having another heart attack are higher than the general population.

A study in rats performed at the Department of Cardiothoracic Surgery, Medical College of Pennsylvania, in Philadelphia, demonstrated the ability of CoQ_{10} to protect the inner lining of arteries from oxidative damage during a simulated heart attack. Rats were treated with CoQ_{10} or placebo before their hearts were subjected to oxygen deprivation. The rats that received the CoQ_{10} tolerated the lack of oxygen better than the control group. Based on the results of this study and others that have shown similar benefits, it would seem prudent for individuals who have angina or are prone to heart attacks to supplement with CoQ_{10}.

Q. If I've just had a heart attack, can CoQ_{10} help increase my chances of surviving longer?

A. Probably. Dr. B. Kuklinski and colleagues, from

the Department of Medicine, Sudstadt Clinic in Rostock, Germany, tested the effects of CoQ$_{10}$ on sixty-one heart-attack patients. These patients were split into two groups. Immediately after hospitalization, members of the first group (thirty-two patients) received a daily dosage of 100 mg of CoQ$_{10}$ and 100 mcg of selenium (a mineral that has antioxidant properties). The control group, consisting of twenty-nine patients, were given placebo (dummy) pills. During the follow-up period of one year, six patients who got the placebo pills were dead from a second heart attack, whereas only one patient from the group that got the antioxidants died—and this patient died from non-cardiac causes. Did CoQ$_{10}$, selenium, or the combination afford the full cardiac protection? We don't know for sure. But considering the natural synergism of antioxidants, the effects of any single antioxidant are magnified by taking additional ones.

Q. What dosage of CoQ$_{10}$ is appropriate in the prevention of heart attacks?

A. My recommended dosage is 30 mg a day. However, make this only one element in your supplement regimen. Take other antioxidants, such as selenium, vitamins E and C, and alpha-lipoic acid.

Q. Is CoQ$_{10}$ helpful for the treatment of arrhythmias?

A. Almost everyone has a temporary episode of an irregular heartbeat manifested as palpitations or a skipped heart beat. Most often, the heart is able to correct itself and go back into a regular rhythm. When these arrhythmias occur more frequently, it's best to see a doctor for a full evaluation. CoQ$_{10}$ may be beneficial in treating arrhythmias by stabilizing the electrical conduction system of the heart. The studies evaluating the role of this nutrient in the prevention of irregular heart rhythms are limited. However, it is reasonable to take 30 mg of CoQ$_{10}$ daily.

Also, if you experience palpitations, I recommend you follow good dietary and lifestyle habits. Excess caffeine, alcohol, and stimulants can make your condition worse. Find ways to reduce stress and get a deep sleep at night. Palpitations occur more frequently after a night of poor sleep. Nutrients such as magnesium, potassium, and fish oils can reduce the risk for heart irregularities as well.

Q. Is CoQ$_{10}$ appropriate if I'm planning to have a heart operation?

A. Yes. CoQ_{10} may reduce the risk of post-surgical complications. During a heart operation, there are times when not enough blood is pumped to the brain, heart, and other tissues. Afterwards, the flow of oxygen-enriched blood resumes. The lack of blood followed by the flooding of oxygen-enriched blood can cause what's called *ischemia/reperfusion injury*, resulting from the excessive formation of free radicals. In my opinion, CoQ_{10} at 30 mg a day, along with other antioxidants, should be recommended by cardiologists before and after performing heart operations.

A study performed on dogs indicates CoQ_{10}'s helpful role. Sixteen dogs were divided into two groups. The first group underwent cardiopulmonary bypass with a temporary stopping of blood flow to the brain. The second group underwent the same procedure, but the dogs were also each given an intravenous dose of 10 mg per kg of body weight of CoQ_{10}. Spinal and brain fluids were removed to study the concentration of free radicals, and the brains of the dogs were also evaluated. The amount of free radicals present in the spinal fluid and the amount of damage to the brain were less in the CoQ_{10} group. The researchers noted, "Oxygen-derived free radicals and abnormal energy metabolism might play critical roles in brain ischemia /reperfusion injury.

Coenzyme Q_{10} could protect the brain by improving cerebral metabolism."

Q. Can CoQ₁₀ help with mitral valve prolapse?

A. There is a valve located in the heart called the *mitral valve* that opens and closes the opening from the left atrium to the left ventricle. Each time the left ventricle beats, the valve closes and blood has only one way to go—that is, through the aorta. When the valve malfunctions and doesn't close well, or actually is pushed back, some of the blood flows back to the atrium. We call this *mitral valve prolapse* or *MVP*. It is a common condition and can be present even in some children. The constant flow of the blood back into the atrium can put pressure on the left ventricle, since it has to keep pumping harder.

In one study, ten patients, ages nine to sixteen years, with MVP and a stressed ventricle received 3 mg of CoQ_{10} per kg (2.2 lbs) of body weight for seven days. Their responses were compared with another group who did not receive the antioxidant. The group on CoQ_{10} showed benefits from CoQ_{10} administration. CoQ_{10} is not a cure for MVP, but in some individuals it can provide a minor benefit.

4.

More Ways
Coenzyme Q_{10}
Can Help

CoQ_{10} is present in every cell in the body. Hence, it is likely that this nutrient can play a role in a diverse number of medical conditions. Previously, I've explained how CoQ_{10} influences cardiovascular conditions. In this chapter, I'll describe some of the CoQ_{10} research in non-cardiovascular areas.

Q. Is CoQ_{10} helpful in fighting breast cancer?

A. Although research with breast cancer and CoQ_{10} is very limited, there is a possibility that this nutrient is helpful. The research published so far certainly is promising. "Partial and complete regression of breast cancer in patients in relation to dosage of coenzyme Q$_{10}$" was the title of an article published by Knud Lockwood, M.D., of Vejle, Denmark, and the late Karl Folkers, Ph.D., of the Institute for Biomedical Research, University of Texas, Austin. When I saw the title of this article, my jaw dropped. Could a natural nutrient actually put a halt to breast cancer?

The study involved thirty-two patients who were given antioxidants (beta-carotene, vitamins C and E, and selenium), essential fatty acids, and 90 mg of CoQ$_{10}$ daily. Six of the thirty-two patients showed partial tumor regression. In one of these six cases, the dosage of CoQ$_{10}$ was increased to 390 mg. In one month, the tumor was no longer palpable (that is, it couldn't be felt). After another month, a mammography confirmed the absence of the tumor.

One may justifiably ask, "How do we know it wasn't the other antioxidants doing the trick and not CoQ$_{10}$?" Well, the researchers did address this question. In the case of this patient, only 90 mg of CoQ$_{10}$ was given during the first year of therapy, and the size of the tumor stabilized at 1.5 to 2 cm (about one-half to three-quarters of an inch) in diameter. The dose was then increased to 390 mg. After two to three months on 390 mg, the tumor regressed. Lockwood and Folkers wrote, "Regression of a tumor of 1.5 to 2 cm in size in up to 3 months on a dosage of 390 mg of CoQ$_{10}$, but not in about 1 year on 90 mg in the same protocol, indicates that CoQ_{10} was dominant in the complete regression of the cancer; and above any benefit from the other nutritional supplements." Lockwood added, "I have treated about two hundred patients with breast cancer a year for thirty-five years, and have never seen a spontaneous regression of a 1.5 to 2 cm breast tumor, and have never seen a comparable regression on any conventional anti-tumor therapy."

Q. Does this mean I should take CoQ_{10} if I have breast cancer?

A. It certainly wouldn't hurt, and it might help. Lockwood's findings are encouraging, and cancer patients should consider adding CoQ_{10} and other antioxidants to their nutritional regimens. However, keep in mind that complete reliance on the results of one study is not wise; sometimes additional studies do not lead to the same outcome. Still, the study discussed in the previous answer is very encouraging. So consider combining CoQ_{10} with other, more accepted therapies for breast cancer.

The nutritional approach to the therapy of cancer has been long neglected by traditional physicians. Over the next few years, we are likely to discover numerous other nutrients that can help in slowing the progression of and/or reversing some cancers.

Q. Is CoQ₁₀ helpful if I'm on chemotherapy?

A. Chemotherapeutic drugs are generally toxins that kill not only tumor cells, but have the ability to damage regular healthy cells, too. Cancer specialists, known as *oncologists*, recognize the potential for normal tissue damage due to chemotherapeutic drugs. Thus, they try to choose drugs that have the most potential in killing cancer cells while leaving the healthy ones near intact. Providing nutrients during chemotherapy can help the healthy cells, but could also help the cancer cells be more resistant to the chemotherapeutic drugs. Therefore, nutritional support during chemotherapy can be a double-edged sword. However, it is important to point out that each type of cancer is different, and each type of chemotherapy is different, too. There are some situations where providing nutrients during chemotherapy can be beneficial.

To put this in perspective, consider a study in which two groups of children with acute lymphoblastic leukemia or non-Hodgkin's lymphoma were treated with chemotherapeutic drugs known as *anthracyclines*. These drugs are known to cause damage to the heart, possibly through a process involving free radicals. The first group of ten patients received 100 mg of CoQ$_{10}$ twice daily, while the second group of ten patients did not. CoQ$_{10}$ was able to protect the heart from damage. The researchers write that "CoQ$_{10}$ given to patients with malignancy during anthracycline therapy is effective in protecting myocardial function from chemotherapeutic cardiotoxicity. Therefore, an associated use of both treatments is suggested for these patients."

If you're on chemotherapeutic drugs, ask your physician if they are toxic to heart tissue. Or, you may ask for a *PDR* (*Physician's Desk Reference*) from the public library and look up the side effects of these chemotherapeutic drugs yourself. If the word *cardiotoxicity* is mentioned, then it may be worthwhile to discuss with your physician the possibility of taking CoQ$_{10}$ to reduce this damage. And please be aware that not all chemotherapeutic drugs damage the heart. Many are harmful to other organs. For instance, *cis-platinum* is known to damage the kidneys.

Q. Can CoQ$_{10}$ protect against toxins or cancer-causing agents?

A. Since it acts as an antioxidant, CoQ$_{10}$ theoretically has the potential to reduce damage from toxins and cancer-causing chemicals. However, research in this area is limited to rodent studies only.

Let me give you an example. Whenever meat is cooked, or overcooked, there is a possibility of cancer-causing agents being formed. One such agent is 2-amino-1-methyl-6-phenylimidazo-pyridine, or PhIP. This toxic chemical damages mitochondria. Rats fed a diet containing 0.2 percent of CoQ_{10} showed the ability to protect against the unfavorable effects of PhIP. It's possible that, in the future, we may find CoQ_{10} to be protective against various other toxins. Let's keep in mind, though, that there are hundreds or thousands of natural compounds in the foods we eat that also have anti-tumor and anti-toxin abilities.

Q. Is CoQ_{10} helpful in chronic fatigue?

A. CoQ_{10} very well may add to your energy, thus reducing the effects of chronic fatigue syndrome. First, let's discuss this condition. Extreme and prolonged tiredness can be caused by a number of medical or psychological conditions. If you constantly feel fatigued, get a thorough physical examination to rule out any serious medical conditions that could account for your lack of energy. Psychological conditions that cause fatigue include depression and anxiety. If your health-care practitioner determines that your fatigue is not due to an obvious medical or psychiatric disorder, it would be worthwhile to try a nutritional approach.

Before diagnosing yourself with chronic fatigue syndrome, I recommend that you review your diet to make sure you are eating the proper balance of protein, fat, and carbohydrate. Some fad diets, such as extreme low-fat, high-carbohydrate diets, can make you tired. I believe it is best to consume a balance of protein, fat, and carbohydrate at each meal. The carbohydrates should come from complex sources such as legumes, whole grains, and vegetables.

You may also benefit from some natural energizers, including herbs such as ginseng; herbal antidepressants such as St. John's wort; and nutrients such as carnitine. Importantly, CoQ$_{10}$ is an excellent energizer, and a dose of 30 to 60 mg in the morning could be helpful. But keep in mind that no nutrient, by itself, is going to be completely effective. Also, mild to moderate physical activity is essential if you want to have more energy. Exercise will help you get a deeper sleep at night. Deep sleep is, by far, one of the best ways to improve energy levels.

Q. Does CoQ$_{10}$ influence degenerative diseases of the brain?

A. Studies evaluating CoQ$_{10}$'s role in preventing and treating brain disorders are limited, but this nutrient may eventually be found to play a positive role in age-related mental decline and certain neurological disorders. For example, an enlightening study was done on *juvenile neuronal ceroid lipofuscinosis* (JNCL), an inherited, progressive neurodegenerative disease. *Lipofuscin* is the term for brown pigment granules that represent lipid fragments associated with age-related wear and tear. Deposits of lipofuscin in the brain naturally occur in many older individuals.

The levels of the antioxidants CoQ_{10} and vitamin E were measured in blood samples of twenty-nine JNCL patients and then compared with forty-eight healthy controls. When compared to controls, significant reduction of the CoQ_{10} level was observed in the JNCL patients. The level of vitamin E was also reduced markedly in JNCL patients. The low levels of CoQ_{10} and vitamin E may link impaired antioxidant protection to this disease. We don't know whether providing CoQ_{10} and vitamin E will help patients with this disorder, but this option should be explored.

Q. Does CoQ_{10} help patients with Parkinson's disease?

A. Researchers at the Veterans Affairs Medical Center, in San Diego, California, have found levels of coenzyme Q_{10} in the mitochondria from Parkinsonian patients to be lower than in mitochondria from age- and sex-matched control subjects. However, limited clinical trials with this nutrient regarding Parkinson's disease have not shown noticeable benefits.

A three-month trial was performed to evaluate the efficacy of 200 mg of CoQ_{10} daily in ten patients with Parkinson's disease. There was no significant effect on the clinical ratings. A year later, another study again did not show any dramatic improvements when 200 mg of CoQ_{10} was administered two, three, or four times per day for one month in fifteen subjects with Parkinson's disease. Oral CoQ_{10} caused a substantial increase in the plasma CoQ_{10} level, but CoQ_{10} did not change the individuals' mean scores on the motor portion of the Unified Parkinson's Disease Rating Scale.

Quite differently, in my experience and in interviews with doctors who use CoQ_{10}, I have heard many reports that CoQ_{10} helps patients with Parkinson's disease have slightly more energy. The jury is still out on the role CoQ_{10} plays in this neurological disorder.

Q. Does CoQ_{10} help treat liver disease?

A. The liver is involved in detoxifying many substances. Its antioxidant reserves may be depleted when it becomes stressed. A Japanese study has shown that patients who have liver disease, whether from hepatitis, cirrhosis, or liver cancer, have a lower amount of antioxidants in their system, including CoQ_{10} and vitamin C. It is not known whether replacing CoQ_{10} will help these patients with their liver problems. However, it is quite possible that other organs and tissues may be undergoing oxidative stress, and the individuals afflicted with these disorders may benefit from CoQ_{10} supplementation. (Keep in mind that excessive alcohol ingestion can place enormous stress on the liver's ability to function properly. A healthy lifestyle is important for proper liver function.)

Q. Does CoQ_{10} play a role in treating thyroid disease?

A. Researchers at the Department of Internal Medicine, Fujita Health University School of Medicine, in Aichi, Japan wanted to clarify the different roles of free radical scavenging systems in various thyroid disorders. They measured the levels of vitamin E and coenzyme Q_{10} in the thyroid tissues of patients with thyroid tumors and Graves' disease. The levels of vitamin E in the thyroid tissue of patients with papillary carcinoma and malignant lymphoma were elevated compared with those in normal thyroid tissues. Conversely, the levels of coenzyme Q_{10} were reduced in the thyroid tissue of patients with Graves' disease and follicular and papillary thyroid carcinomas. The researchers wrote, "These findings imply that vitamin E and coenzyme Q_{10} as antioxidants play some role in thyroid follicular cell function." The practical applications of these findings are not clear at this time. I would expect that a small amount of CoQ_{10}, such as 10 mg, would be safe to ingest in patients with thyroid disease.

Q. Can CoQ_{10} treat vitiligo?

A. *Vitiligo* is a skin disorder associated with healthy looking skin except for areas and patches of no pigmentation. The condition is thought to involve an autoimmune process. But oxidation and, therefore, CoQ_{10} may play roles in this condition. There has been only one study evaluating levels of CoQ_{10} in the skin of patients with vitiligo.

To examine the sensitivity of vitiligo melanocytes (skin cells involved in pigmentation) to external oxidative stress, researchers at San Gallicano Dermatologic Institute in Rome, Italy, studied antioxidants in cultured melanocytes of normal subjects and in melanocytes from apparently normal skin of vitiligo patients. The activity of natural antioxidants such as superoxide dismutase and catalase, and the concentrations of vitamin E and CoQ_{10} in the skin cells, were evaluated in cell cultures. In addition, cells were exposed to various concentrations of an oxidizing agent. Compared to normal melanocytes, vitiligo melanocytes showed low levels of CoQ_{10}, but higher or normal levels of other antioxidants. Furthermore, vitiligo mela-nocytes were susceptible to the toxic effect of the oxidant. The researchers wrote, "Our results demonstrate the presence of an imbalance in the anti-oxidant system in vitiligo melanocytes and provide further support for a free radical-mediated damage as an initial pathogenic event in melanocyte degeneration in vitiligo."

Whether supplying CoQ_{10} to patients with vitiligo will be of benefit is currently not known. However, supplementing with 10 to 30 mg a day may be worthwhile. The antioxidant capabilities of the nutrient are promising.

Q. Is CoQ$_{10}$ helpful in preventing and/or treating gum disease?

A. If you don't floss or brush your teeth, your gin-giva—the tissue around your teeth—eventually will recede, get inflamed, and possibly even bleed. Inflammation of the gingiva is known as *gingivitis*. If the gingivitis gets worse, teeth may loosen. At this more severe stage, the condition is referred to as *periodontitis*.

I was surprised when I first heard that CoQ$_{10}$ had a role to play in the therapy of periodontitis. It turns out that the gingival tissue, like the heart, has sub-stantial energy requirements. Apparently, CoQ$_{10}$ plays an important role in energy metabolism in gin-gival tissue. A few studies have shown that CoQ$_{10}$ administration can counter periodontal inflamma-tion. It's also been found that applying CoQ$_{10}$, dis-persed in oil, to actual inflamed gingival sites in the mouth can improve periodontal symptoms.

Not every scientist accepts that CoQ$_{10}$ is beneficial in periodontitis. Dr. K. Watts, from the Department of Periodontology and Preventive Dentistry, Guy's Hospital, London, expressed his skepticism in the *British Dental Journal*. He wrote that a "review of the available literature does not give any ground for the claims made, and CoQ$_{10}$ has no place in periodontal treatment." It is evident that scientists don't always agree on every issue. It will take more research to resolve the CoQ_{10}/periodontitis issue. In the meantime, keep in mind that no amount of CoQ_{10} will replace the need to brush and floss teeth regularly, and periodic dental cleaning by a hygenist is extremely important.

Q. Is CoQ_{10} involved in the health of sperm?

A. CoQ_{10} is present at high levels in human seminal fluid (semen), which is needed to transport sperm. It appears that CoQ_{10} serves an antioxidant function protecting semen from oxidative damage. This is extremely important since semen carries DNA to the female's egg for fertilization. Damage to DNA can result in a failure to conceive or in fetal abnormalities.

In patients with *varicocele*, which is kind of like a varicose vein in the testicles, CoQ_{10} is present in lower amounts. Scientists at the Institute of Endocrinology, Catholic University School of Medicine, Rome, Italy, have noted that since "coenzyme Q_{10} is an antioxidant molecule involved in the defense of the cell from free radical damage, high concentrations of CoQ$_{10}$ is seminal fluid may represent a mechanism of protection of the spermatozoa. In varicocele patients, this mechanism could be deficient, leading to higher sensitivity to oxidative damage." At this time we don't know whether supplementation with CoQ$_{10}$ can help patients with varicocele have healthier sperm. But this is an intri-guing possibility.

Q. Is CoQ$_{10}$ beneficial to athletes?

A. Many individuals who take CoQ$_{10}$ notice an increase in energy. I have personally experienced this effect. Would administering CoQ$_{10}$ help athletes during intense training? As of now, research finds no beneficial results from CoQ$_{10}$.

Researchers at the Department of Physiology and Pharmacology, Karolinska Institute, Stockholm, Sweden, investigated the effects of oral supplementation of CoQ$_{10}$ in nine individuals, compared with a placebo, on aerobic and anaerobic physical performance over twenty-two days. The supplementation period included five days of high intensity anaerobic training between the eleventh and fourteenth days. The results demonstrated that on an anaerobic cycling test, the placebo group showed a significantly greater improvement than the CoQ10-

group after a supplementation and training period. Further, the CoQ$_{10}$ group had a significantly lower increase in total work performed during the seven training sessions, compared with the placebo group. There was a significant increase in maximal blood lactate accumulation during cycling in the both groups, when compared with levels before the training and recovery period. The researchers concluded that for high-intensity anaerobic training, CoQ$_{10}$ was not of benefit, and in fact, the placebo group performed better.

Based on this one study, it appears that in normal, healthy athletes, CoQ$_{10}$ cannot be counted on to improve performance. Additional studies are needed to confirm or dispute these findings.

5.

Taking Coenzyme Q_{10} Supplements

Chances are, when you go to a health food store, pharmacy, or other retail outlet, you will find a number of different CoQ_{10} products with different dosages. You will also encounter dozens of different vitamins, herbs, amino acids, hormones, and other nutrients on the shelves that you might consider taking. How do you know which CoQ_{10} product to purchase and whether the combination with your other supplements is appropriate? As with any nutrient, the dosage and timing can make a significant influence on the therapeutic response. This chapter discusses these practical matters.

Q. In what forms and dosages are CoQ_{10} supplements available?

A. CoQ$_{10}$ is available in oil-filled capsules, powder-filled hardshell capsules, powder-based tablets, chewable wafers, and a solubilized form. There are dozens of vitamin companies that sell this nutrient. The capsules range from 10 to 100 mg, although 30 mg seems to be the most common dosage. You will also find this nutrient added to some multivitamin tablets in dosages ranging from 5 to 30 mg.

Q. What dosage should I take?

A. There are yet no guidelines set by doctors on the optimal dosage of CoQ$_{10}$ and many opinions are available. I recommend that my healthy middle-aged and older patients take about 10 mg a day. So if your health-care professional and you have decided to add CoQ$_{10}$ to your overall regimen, start with a low dose of 10 mg in the morning. I always feel that most medicines and nutrients should be started conservatively. Over my many years of practice as a physician, I have realized that there are individuals who are extremely sensitive to supplements and react to them even if minute dosages are used. By starting low, we minimize any potential adverse effects.

If you have symptoms of heart disease and find

that they are not improving after you've been on 10 mg for a few days, you can increase the dose to 10 mg twice daily for another few days. If your heart symptoms improve, you can stay at this dosage. If not, gradually increase your dose by 10 mg every few days, until satisfactory results have been achieved.

Q. How well is CoQ_{10} absorbed?

A. In 1997, scientists at the Technical University in Lyngby, Denmark, administered 30 mg of CoQ_{10} as a pill to volunteers and then proceeded to measure blood levels. They also gave another group of people cooked pork heart that contained 30 mg of CoQ_{10}. They wanted to see if there was any difference between giving the CoQ_{10} in a capsule versus food. The increase in the blood-CoQ_{10} levels reached a maximum six hours after ingestion of either the capsules or the meal. Both the capsule and the pork were able to raise blood levels significantly. The researchers commented that this "study indicates that CoQ_{10} present in the diet may contribute significantly to plasma (blood) CoQ_{10} concentrations in man."

We should also keep in mind that the type of formulation the CoQ$_{10}$ is mixed with can influence its absorption. One study has shown that CoQ$_{10}$ dissolved in soybean oil was a good way to ingest this nutrient. This makes sense because CoQ$_{10}$ is fat-soluble. Therefore, ingesting it with a meal is an appropriate way to supplement with this nutrient. It is quite likely that formulating CoQ$_{10}$ with any number of oils would be effective in terms of its absorption.

The absorption rate of different products on the market can vary. A study sponsored by a company that manufactures the solubilized form has found their product to be better absorbed. In my judgment, companies selling CoQ$_{10}$ products should provide absorption test results on request.

Q. What are normal blood levels of CoQ$_{10}$?

A. A high level of CoQ$_{10}$ is normally found in the bloodstream, estimated to be 0.1 mg per 100 ml of blood. When volunteer subjects were given 30 mg of CoQ$_{10}$ three times daily, their levels rose from 0.1 mg to 2 mg. This level remained steady for the duration of the study, which was nine months. After stopping the nutrient, blood levels returned to normal.

Q. Does CoQ$_{10}$ have side effects?

A. Fortunately, CoQ$_{10}$ has few side effects, and most of these occur only at high dosages. In a study conducted in Italy, 2,664 patients with congestive heart failure were given an average of 100 mg CoQ$_{10}$ for a period of three months (Baggio, 1994). Only 36 patients out of 2,664 (1.5 percent) reported side effects. The most common was nausea, which occurred in thirty patients. This rate of side effects is very low. And at the end of the study, the results indicated that at least two-thirds of the patients improved. Most common benefits noted were a decrease in edema, lung congestion, shortness of breath, and palpitations.

In another study, doses ranging form 75 to 600 mg a day were given to more than 400 patients with a variety of different heart problems. The average length of time CoQ$_{10}$ was given was a year and a half. No apparent side effects were noted from CoQ$_{10}$ administration except for rare cases of nausea.

Anecdotally, I have come across several side effects of CoQ$_{10}$. Some individuals report a feeling of over-stimulation on doses higher than 60 mg. Insomnia can occur if too-high doses are taken, even in the morning. No serious adverse effects have been reported from experiments using daily supplements of up to 200 mg of CoQ$_{10}$ for six to twelve months, and 100 mg daily for up to six years.

Q. For how long can I take CoQ$_{10}$?

A. As noted previously, this nutrient has been given to patients for many years without any noticeable side effects. Presently, there is no cause to worry about taking CoQ$_{10}$ for an extended period of time. If you have heart disease, and CoQ$_{10}$ is helping you, then you may need to take this nutrient indefinitely. Your doctor or nutritionist can work with you to find the best dosages. As with any kind of supplement or drug, just take the lowest dose that works.

Q. What do people feel when they take CoQ$_{10}$?

A. Patients who take CoQ$_{10}$ most often have positive responses. As a rule, the effect from 30 mg is subtle, mostly consisting of a slightly higher energy level. When dosages are increased to 60 mg or higher, people notice an increase in energy as the day progresses, with an urge to be more physically active. Many patients report a slight mood elevation with enhanced focus and motivation, along with the desire to engage in conversation. The 90- or 120-mg dose, though, can be too much for some patients since it can lead to excessive stimulation and alertness well into late evening when it's time to slow down and get ready for sleep.

Q. Do healthy individuals need to take CoQ_{10}?

A. The body is able to make small amounts of CoQ_{10}. This, along with dietary intake, seems to fulfill the body's demands for CoQ_{10} in younger, healthy individuals. However, as we get older, the body may not be able to make as much CoQ_{10} and supplementation can prove to be beneficial.

If you're the type of person who consumes a lot of oils, such as from salad dressings, or if you take large doses of supplemental fish oils, consider the protective role of CoQ_{10}. Twenty-two healthy young subjects were given supplements of fish oils and then had their blood measured for lipid oxidation, along with vitamin E and C levels. CoQ_{10} was found to prevent lipid peroxidation and also was able to spare vitamin E degradation. However, other studies have not indicated that ingesting fish oils lead to oxidation.

Q. Can CoQ₁₀ be combined with carnitine to improve heart function?

A. Yes. There are several nutrients that improve heart function. One particular one that shows a great deal of promise is *carnitine*, a naturally occurring compound found in most cells in the body, particularly the brain and neural tissues, muscles, heart, and testicles. Carnitine plays a crucial role in muscle function, and studies have found carnitine supplementation at 2 grams a day to improve aerobic capacity in athletes.

Carnitine can be obtained from the diet, particularly animal foods. Most non-vegetarians consume about 100 to 300 mg of carnitine a day, and the body is able to synthesize this nutrient from the amino acids lysine and methionine if dietary intake is inadequate. Vitamins B_3, B_6, and C help the process of carnitine manufacture in the liver and kidneys. Carnitine helps shuttle fatty acids and two carbon acetyl groups located in heart-muscle cells into the mitochondria for energy production. The fatty acids cannot cross the mitochondrial cell membrane without carnitine. Supplementing with this nutrient can be helpful, and combining it with CoQ₁₀ is not dangerous.

Q. What about combining CoQ₁₀ with other antioxidant nutrients and hormones?

A. More and more research is accumulating about the positive interrelationship between different antioxidants. I'm becoming increasingly convinced that it is wiser to take small amounts of a variety of antioxidants rather than a high amount of one or two. Each antioxidant has a different role in the body, and they can often complement each other.

As we age, our body's antioxidant system does not work as well and our antioxidant requirements increase. In addition to eating a variety of fresh fruits and vegetables, which contain hundreds of flavonoid and carotenoid antioxidants, you may wish to add the following antioxidants to your regimen: vitamin E, between 100 and 200 mg, once a day; vitamin C, between 100 to 500 mg, twice a day; CoQ₁₀, 10 to 20 mg, once a day; alpha-lipoic acid, 10 to 20 mg, once a day; and selenium, 50 to 100 mcg, once a day.

Q. Will CoQ₁₀ combine poorly with melatonin?

A. CoQ$_{10}$ should not interact with the use of melatonin. Most often, CoQ$_{10}$ is taken in the morning or during the day, whereas melatonin is used at night for sleep. So you have no reason to feel that you cannot take both.

Q. Are there any studies done on DHEA and CoQ$_{10}$?

A. One concern that has been raised with the use of DHEA (dehydroepiandrosterone, the adrenal hormone) is that in rats given excessively high dosages, liver damage has occurred. This liver damage is extremely rare in humans and does not occur in the dosages normally used for hormone replacement. In a 1997 study, when rats were given 300 mg of DHEA per kg along with CoQ$_{10}$, the damage to the liver was minimal. Whether this finding has any relevance to humans is not clear at this time. But why not take precautionary measures? It certainly wouldn't hurt for anyone who is taking DHEA to take a small amount of CoQ$_{10}$.

Q. Can I combine heart medicines with CoQ$_{10}$?

A. Yes, they can be combined, but with some caution and, ideally, under the supervision of your physician. Because CoQ$_{10}$ strengthens the heart muscle, it may reduce requirements of prescription heart stimulations. Adjusting dosages in this situation is best left to a physician.

In addition, remember that there are dozens of heart medicines, including different types of diuretics (water pills), anti-arrhythmic agents (to prevent heart irregularities), blood pressure medicines (calcium channel blockers, blood vessel dilators), digitalis, and others. Studies evaluating the combination of CoQ$_{10}$ and these various medicines have not been done. It becomes even more complicated when CoQ$_{10}$ is used with multiple medicines. Therefore, consult your health-care provider. Any changes made in the dosages of medicines, and the addition of CoQ$_{10}$ to your regimen should be done in a gradual, step-by-step way.

Q. Are there any cautions when combining CoQ$_{10}$ with blood thinners?

A. There's always a possibility that nutrients can interact with pharmaceutical medicines. This is why you should discuss supplementation with your physician anytime you plan to add nutrients to your regimen when you are currently taking other drugs. Drug interaction between coenzyme Q_{10} and *warfarin*, a blood thinner, has been reported. Warfarin is often prescribed for people who clot very easily. Medical conditions that can result from clots include heart attacks, strokes, and pulmonary embolism (when a clot travels to the lungs).

A patient history is recorded in a medical journal of a female of seventy-two years of age who was treated with warfarin. She showed less responsiveness to warfarin than previously. It appeared she had taken coenzyme Q_{10}, and when this was stopped, her responsiveness to warfarin was the same as before. Patients in treatment with warfarin should be aware of the possible risk of treatment failure when taking coenzyme Q_{10}.

Q. Could CoQ_{10} be considered an anti-aging nutrient?

A. Based on the research and clinical experiences of physicians, CoQ_{10} results in improved heart function—the heart works as if it were younger. Most of the studies, though, involved sick people who had considerable room for improvement. So far, there have not been any studies giving CoQ_{10} to healthy people for many years and then checking to see if taking this nutrient helped the participants to be healthier and to live longer.

A study with laboratory rats did not show CoQ_{10} to extend their life spans. I need to mention, though, that there are always problems in interpreting rodent studies in terms of their significance to humans. Humans often respond differently to supplements than do rodents. Furthermore, it's very hard to translate the dose given to a rat to the equivalent dose in humans. Determining this by weight ratio can be very misleading. An additional point to keep in mind is that the same nutrient can have beneficial, neutral, or harmful effects depending on the dosage used.

Conclusion

There is little doubt that CoQ_{10} can be beneficial in combating cardiovascular diseases, especially chronic heart failure. Its capacity to contribute to healthy cellular-energy production is clear. As this book explains, CoQ_{10} may also play a role in enhancing the immune system and perhaps may even help the body fight certain types of cancer. As with many other nutrients currently available, extensive studies must be conducted to determine the ideal dosages and how we can best use this important nutrient.

The published evidence on CoQ_{10}'s ability to be beneficial in improving heart function, and the fact that it is a very good antioxidant, have persuaded me, for now, that small amounts of this nutrient may provide some preventive benefits. I'm currently taking 10 mg most days, and if I ever were diagnosed with cancer or heart disease, I would increase my dosage. There are days, though, that I skip taking my supplements. It's just a personal preference, just in case an imbalance of nutrients is occurring.

To reap the already-known advantages of CoQ$_{10}$, talk to your health-care professional about starting supplementation. Follow the conservative dosage plan suggested in Chapter 5. You'll be surprised at how CoQ$_{10}$ can change your life for the better!

Glossary

Amino acid. A molecule that contains nitrogen and serves as a unit of structure for proteins.

Antioxidant. A substance that combines with free radicals, neutralizes them, and thus prevents the deterioration of DNA, RNA, lipids, and proteins. Vitamins C, E, and beta-carotene are the best known antioxidants, but more and more are being discovered each year.

Atherosclerosis. A condition in which the arteries in the heart and other parts of the body accumulate plaque and become narrow, decreasing the flow of blood and increasing the risk of a clot. It's also known as "hardening of the arteries."

ATP (adenosine triphosphate). The primary energy currency of a cell, derived from the metabolism of glucose, amino acids, and fatty acids.

Cell. The smallest organized unit of living structure in the body. There are trillions of cells in humans; the brain alone has close to one trillion cells. The body's tissues are composed of many cells.

Cell membrane. A thin layer, consisting mostly of fatty acids, that surrounds each cell and regulates what enters and exits that cell.

Cholesterol. The most abundant steroid in animal tissues. It is present in some of the animal foods we eat. Our liver can also make cholesterol if there's not enough in our diet. Cholesterol is used to make steroid hormones.

Coenzyme. A substance that is either necessary for the normal function of, or enhances the activity of, an enzyme. Several vitamins act as coenzymes.

Free radical. A molecule that lacks an electron and aggressively seeks to replace it. Free radicals can do damage to cells by pairing with other molecules, causing oxidation. Free radicals change the normal functioning of cells.

Lipoproteins. Compounds that contain lipids and proteins. Almost all of the lipids in blood, including cholesterol, are transported as lipoprotein complexes. The two best-known of the many lipoproteins in the blood are HDL (high-density lipoproteins, the "good" cholesterol) and LDL (low-density lipoproteins, the "bad" cholesterol).

Metabolism. The chemical and physical processes continuously occurring in the body, involving the creation and breakdown of molecules. For instance, glucose can be metabolized to release its energy as ATP.

Mitochondria. The chemical factories of cells, where energy is made. Hundreds of mitochondria are present in each cell.

Molecule. The smallest possible combination of atoms that retains the chemical properties of the substance. For instance, a molecule of water consists of three atoms: two are hydrogen, and one is oxygen.

Oxidant. A substance, such as a free radical, that causes oxidation.

Oxidation. The process by which a compound reacts with oxygen and loses an electron.

Placebo. A dummy pill that contains no active ingredient.

Platelet. A small round or oval cell found in the blood and involved in blood clotting.

References

The information in this book is drawn from many scientific references. Below are listed some of those references.

Aberg F, Appelkvist EL, Broijersen A, Eriksson M, Angelin B, Hjemdahl P, Dallner G, "Gemfibrozil-induced decrease in serum ubiquinone and alpha- and gamma- tocopherol levels in men with combined hyperlipidaemia," *Eur J Clin Invest* 28 (1998), 3: 235–242.

Baggio E, Gandini R, Plancher AC, Passeri M, Carmosino G, "Italian multicenter study on the safety and efficacy of coenzyme Q_{10} as adjunctive therapy in heart failure," *Molec Asp Med* 15 (1994): S287–294.

Chopra RK, Goldman R, Sinatra ST, Bhagavan HN, "Relative bioavailability of coenzyme Q_{10} formulations in human subjects," *Internat J Vit Nutr Res* 68 (1998), 2: 109–113.

Crane FL, Haten Y, Lester RI, Widmer C, "Isolation of a quinone from the beef heart mitochondria," *Biochim Biophys Acta* 25 (1957): 220–221.

De Pinieux G, Chariot P, Ammi-Salid M, Louarn F, Lejonc JL, et al., "Lipid-lowering drugs and mitochondrial function: effects of HMG_CoA reductase inhibitors on serum ubiquinone and blood lactate/pyruvate ratio," *Br J Clin Pharmacol* 42 (1996): 333–337.

Digiesi V, Cantini F, Oradel, et al., "Coenzyme Q_{10} in essential hypertension," *Molec Aspects Med* 15 (1994): S257–263.

Folkers K, Moesgaard S, Morita M, "A one year bioavailability study of CoQ_{10} with 3 months withdrawal period," *Molec Aspects Med* 15 (1994): S281–285.

Hallstrom H, "Oskadlighetsbedomning av coenzym Q_{10}," *Var Foda* 45 (1993): 250–259.

Hanioka T, Tanaka M, Ojima M, Shizukuishi S, Folkers K, "Effect of topical application of CoQ_{10} on adult periodontitis," *Molec Aspect Med* 15 (1994): S241–248.

Khan S, Nyce J, "Effects of ubiquinone and meval-onic acid on hepatic peroxisomal enzymes induced by dehydroepiandrosterone," *Pharm Toxicol* 80 (1997): 118–121.

Lagendijk J, Ubbink JB, et al., "Ubiquinol /Ubiquinone ratio as marker of oxidative stress in coronary artery disease," *Res Comm Mol Path Pharm* 95 (1997), 1: 11–18.

Landbo C, Almdal TP, "Interaction between war-farin and coenzyme Q10," *Ugeskr Laeger* 160 (May 25, 1998), 22: 3226–3227.

Langsjoen H, Langsjoen P, Langsjoen P, Willis R, Folkers K, "Usefulness of CoQ10 in clinical cardiol-ogy: A long-term study," *Molec Aspects Med* 15 (1994): S165–175.

Langsjoen P, Langsjoen P, Willis R, Folkers K, "Treatment of essential hypertension with CoQ_{10}," *Molec Aspects Med* 15 (1994): S265–272.

Lockwood K, Moesgaard S, Folkers K, "Partial and complete regression of breast cancer in patients in relation to dosage of coenzyme Q_{10}," *Biochem Biophys Res Commun* 199 (1994): 1504–1508.

Lonnrot K, Mets-Ketela T, Alho H, "The role of coenzyme Q10 in aging: a follow-up study on life-long oral supplementation in rats," *Gerontology* 41 (1995), suppl 2: 109–120.

Malm C, Svensson M, Ekblom B, Sjodin B, "Effects of ubiquinone-10 supplementation and high intensity training on physical performance in humans," *Acta Physiol Scand* 161 (Nov 1997), 3: 379–384.

Mancini A, Conte G, Milardi D, De Marinis L, Littarru GP, "Relationship between sperm cell ubiquinone and seminal parameters in subjects with and without varicocele," *Andrologia* 30 (1998), 1: 1–4

Mano T, Iwase K, Hayashi R, Hayakawa N, et al., "Vitamin E and coenzyme Q concentrations in the thyroid tissues of patients with various thyroid disorders," *Am J Med Sci* 315 (1998), 4: 230–232.

Maresca V, Roccella M, Roccella F, et al., "Increased sensitivity to peroxidative agents as a possible pathogenic factor of melanocyte damage in vitiligo," *J Invest Dermatol* 109 (1997), 3: 310–313.

McRee JT, Hanioka T, Shizukuishi S, Folkers K, "Therapy with CoQ10 for patients with periodontal disease. Effect of CoQ10 on subgingival microorganisms," *J Dent Health* 43 (1993): 659–666.

Mohr D, Bowry VW, Stocker R, "Dietary supplementation with CoQ10 results in increased levels of Ubiquinol-10 within circulating lipoproteins and increased resistance of human low-density lipoprotein to the initiation of lipid peroxidation," *Biochim Biophys Acta* 1126 (1992): 247–254.

Morisco C, Nappi A, Argenziano D, et al., "Noninvasive evaluation of cardiac hemodynamics during exercise in patients with chronic heart failure: effects of short-term CoQ10 treatment," *Molec Aspects Med* 15 (1994): S155–163.

Oda T, "Recovery of load-induced left ventricular diastolic dysfunction by CoQ10 echocardiographic study," *Molec Aspects Med* 15 (1994): S149–154.

Overvad OK, Diamant B, Holm L, Holmer G, Mortensen SA, Stender S, "Efficacy and safety of dietary supplementation containing Q_{10}," *Ugeskr Laeger* 159 (1997), 15: 7309–7315.

Porter DA, Costill DL, Zachwieja JJ, et al., "The effect of oral CoQ_{10} on the exercise tolerance of middle-aged, untrained men," Int J Sports Med 16 (1995): 421–427.

Shults CW, Beal MF, Fontaine D, Nakano K, Haas RH, "Absorption, tolerability, and effects on mitochondrial activity of oral coenzyme Q$_{10}$ in parkinsonian patients," *Neurology* 50 (1998), 3: 793–795.

Soja AM, Mortensen SA, "Treatment of chronic cardiac insufficiency with coenzyme Q$_{10}$, results of meta-analysis in controlled clinical trials," Ugeskr Laeger 159 (1997), 49: 7302–7308.

Stocker R, Bowry VW, Frei B, Ubiquinol-10 protects human low density lipoprotein more efficiently against lipid peroxidation than does alph-tocopherol," *Proc Natl Acad Sci USA* 88 (1991): 1646–1650.

Sugiyama S, Yamada K, Haykawa M, et al., "Effects of ubiquinone-enriched diet on deterioration of mitochondrial respiratory function caused by fried beef derived mutagenic factor in rats," *Biochem Mol Biol Int* 40 (1996): 305–314.

Swart I, Rossouw J, Lot JM, Kruger MC, "The effect of L-carnitine on plasma carnitine levels and various performance parameters of male marathon athletes," *Nutrition Research* 17 (1997), 3: 405–414.

Thomas SR, Neuzil J, Stocker R, "Cosupplementation with Coenzyme Q prevents the prooxidant effect of alpha-tocopherol and increases the resistance of LDL to transition metal-dependent oxidation initiation," *Arterioscler Thromb Vasc Biol* 16 (1996): 687–696.

Watts T, "Coenzyme Q_{10} and periodontal treatment: is there any beneficial effect?" *Br Dental J* 178 (1995): 209–213.

Weber C, Jakobsen TS, Mortensen SA, et al., "Antioxidative effect of dietary coenzyme Q_{10} in human blood plasma," *International Journal Vitamin Nutrition Research* 64 (1994): 311–315.

Weber C, Bysted A, Helmer G, "Intestinal absorption of CoQ_{10} administered in a meal or as capsules to healthy subjects," *Nutrition Research* 6 (1997), vol 17: 941–945.

Weis M, Mortenseri SA, Rassing MR, et al., "Bioavailability of four oral CoQ10 formulations in healthy volunteers," *Molec Aspects Med* 15 (1994): S273–280.

Yamamoto Y, et al., "Oxidative stress in patients with hepatitis, cirrhosis, and hepatoma evaluated by plasma antioxidants," *Biochem Biophys Res Commun* 247 (June 9, 1998), 1: 166–170.

Yokohama H, Lingle D, Crestanello JA, Kamelgard J, et al., "Coenzyme Q_{10} protects coronary endothelial function from ischemia reperfusion injury via an antioxidant effect," *Surgery* 120 (1996): 189–196.

Zhen R, Wenxiang D, Zhaokang S, et al., "Mechanisms of brain injury with deep hypothermic circulatory arrest and protective effects of coenzyme Q_{10}," *J Thorac Cardiovasc Surg* 108 (1994): 126–133.

Suggested Readings

Bliznakov EG and Hunt L. *The Miracle Nutrient: Coenzyme Q_{10}.* New York: Bantam Books, 1986.

Heber D. *Natural Remedies for a Healthy Heart.* Garden City Park, N.Y: Avery Publishing Group, 1998.

Index